From Widowmaker To LVAD To Heart Transplant

Twelve Miracles of Faith

By: James Clifton (Jimmy) Davis

Preface: About the Author

James Clifton (Jimmy) Davis is retired and currently resides near the small town of Swansea, South Carolina, United States. He served as senior pastor for churches in Indiana and South Carolina. Jimmy was educated at Charleston Southern University, Charleston, South Carolina, The Southern Baptist Theological Seminary, Louisville, Kentucky, and Trinity Theological Seminary, Newburgh, Indiana. Jimmy's prayer is that you will gain God's great comfort from reading this very real story of his life; from the time of just over a year before he suffered a widow maker heart attack to the time of transition, living with the HeartMate Series Three LVAD heart pump, and moving forward to a heart transplant on December 17, 2020.

Introduction: A note from Jimmy

During my ministry years I have written fifty-two books, which are printed in many of the languages of the world, and distributed for sale on the Internet. These books are available in printed form, or e-books, and were written to help church leaders and Christians in individual and group ministry. These books can be found by doing a Google search for Jimmy Davis books. I have also owned three businesses during my life, which include an auto parts store with a full service automotive garage; a restaurant at Myrtle Beach, SC; and an Internet sales store. At the time of this writing I am 69 years old, enjoy spending time with family, friends, and tinkering with wristwatches, clocks, antique tools, and auto mechanics. I also help my cousin with estate sales. My intention for writing this short story is to help those people who either currently have, or are considering upcoming surgery for an LVAD, or a heart transplant. If you are currently waiting for an LVAD, please do not be afraid! This surgery, although indeed major, will most likely improve your overall health, and allow you to continue to live, and do many of the things in life you have always enjoyed. If you already have an LVAD, then perhaps you can identify with me in many aspects that we both may share; because we were willing to take the chance to receive a blessing that would improve our health. I am very thankful to all of the professionals serving in the medical fields as well as my family members and friends for a tremendous amount of support I have received. I have truly been blessed more than I ever can imagine, and certainly more than I deserve. May God also bless you in whatever stage of health you currently endure. Always look toward the future with anticipation that great things can and will happen; and may we always be thankful together for each and every day for the blessings of life.

Miracle Number One:

As I begin this short story of the last few years of my life, I must back up in my time line to November 1, 2017, to tell about this miracle of full blessing in my life before I suffered the widow maker heart attack. My cousin Carolyn and I were finishing an estate sale in the Irmo, South Carolina area. She owns a liquidation company, and I have helped her with this since the beginning of the start-up of her company about eight years. All day long I had been going to the bathroom to urinate while we were running the sale, with very little results. Every time I would attempt to urinate, only a tablespoon amount of urine would flow out, and I was growing more and more miserable, and also getting very irritable. As the day wore on, I became more and more uncomfortable and figured that a kidney stone may be the problem. I had been able to pass three kidney stones in the past and, even though it had been about twenty years since I passed the last one, I was somewhat familiar with what was happening to my body. I've always tried to be in tune to what happens to my body but this time felt just a bit different, so I wasn't totally sure I was suffering from a kidney stone. When we got in the car to go home, I commented that I didn't believe I could drive home. My cousin, Carolyn, indicated to me that if she were driving, she would take me straight to the emergency room to see what was wrong with me. I thought my problem was a kidney stone, but didn't know just how severe it would be. I said, "Let's just go buy three cold beers, and I'll just go home and drink the beer and take a few AZO Standard pills to relax my bladder." I had done this when I was about 40 years old, it worked well, and I had passed a kidney stone about the size of a bb without too much difficulty. We made the correct decision and decided to go the emergency room instead. Had I drank the beer and taken AZO Standard, I might not have survived. Upon arrival at the emergency room at Lexington Medical Center, the nurse checked my blood pressure and it was super high: 238/190. I was immediately rushed to an exam room in the ER and given an IV in my arm to bring my blood pressure down. Within a few hours, I was taken to the CT scan room. I had already told the attendants and doctor

I felt sure my problem was a kidney stone. It was indeed a kidney stone, the size of a ping pong ball, a "boulder", as the doctor later stated, and it had already dropped out of my left kidney, and was resting on the top of the ureter. There were also four other small stones found in my left kidney, and one small kidney stone in my right kidney. All of these were found during the CT scan. The ping pong size kidney stone was sitting on top of the tube going to my bladder, the ureter; and had almost fully stopping the urine flow. After a few hours of rest in the emergency room, when my blood pressure was down to almost normal, I was discharged. An appointment was set for me to see a kidney surgeon a few days later. For the next few days, I would have to try to urinate about every twenty to thirty minutes, with very little results. This went on 24/7; just praying I would soon get some relief.

How would I get through this? I had a wedding for a family member I had promised to officiate at 701 Whaley Street in Columbia, South Carolina on November 4th, 2017, only 3 days after the verdict of a boulder size kidney stone in my left kidney. Well, I put on my official black robe for the wedding event, and with God's help, I made it through the wedding ceremony without any problems at all. God is good, and you can always depend on His grace in all your times of need.

My kidney doctor scheduled lithotripsy, a treatment, using ultrasound shock waves, by which a kidney stone is broken into small particles that can be passed out by the body, or collected in a small basket and pulled out of the body through the penis during the lithotripsy surgery. Lithotripsy is a medical procedure involving the physical destruction of hardened masses like kidney stones, and is a term derived from the Greek words meaning "breaking (or pulverizing) stones." After my first treatment, I asked my doctor how much of the kidney stone he was able to remove. He said, "None! I just managed to crack the big one up a little bit." After seven total hours of out patient lithotripsy surgery, five times of being put to sleep, five times and going to the operation room at the hospital, the large kidney stone and the four other smaller kidney stones in my left kidney were gone. I still had the small kidney stone in my right kidney. All of this took place over a period of over two months. What a journey, but still, at the end, what a relief!

    During the next visit to my kidney specialist doctor for a follow-up appointment, he indicated to me that I was still retaining about one liter of urine in my bladder at all times. I had an enlarged prostrate. My doctor indicated that a surgery called TURP would be the final answer to my problems. Transurethral resection of the prostate (commonly known as a TURP) is a fairly common urological operation. The surgeon reaches the prostate by putting an instrument into the end of the penis and through the urethra. This instrument, called a resectoscope, is about 12 inches long, and .5 inch in diameter. It contains a lighted camera and valves that control irrigating fluid. It also contains an electrical wire loop that cuts tissue and seals blood vessels. The wire loop is guided by the surgeon to remove the tissue blocking the urethra one piece at a time. The pieces of tissue are carried by the irrigating fluid into the bladder, and then flushed out at the end of the procedure. It is used to treat benign prostatic hyperplasis (BPH). As the name indicates, it is performed by visualizing the prostate through the urethra, and removing tissue by electrocautery, or sharp dissection. This is considered the most effective treatment for BPH. This procedure is done with general anesthetic. A triple lumen catheter is inserted through the urethra to irrigate and drain the bladder after the surgical procedure is complete. This catheter remained in me for eight miserable days, with a bag of bloody urine strapped to my lower leg that I had to empty every few hours. The procedure worked for me, but was not a walk in the park as some claim it to be. About two months after the TURP surgery, I passed the small kidney stone that was in my right kidney. My urine flow was finally back to normal, and the best it had been in over twenty years.

The reason I am indicating that the kidney stones and the TURP surgery was miracle number one is because after looking back in hindsight, if these health issues were not addressed before the widowmaker heart attack on December 2, 2018, I probably would not have survived. Because I went to the hospital believing I had a kidney stone, I was placed on blood pressure medication. Had I not been on blood pressure medication, I could have possibly had a stroke or even died from the heart attack I was to have on December 2, 2018. Again, God is good, and He blessed me with eliminating these problems before the heart attack. Anyone can find a blessing in even the worst circumstance. God is good, even when people are not! The summer of 2018 was great. I felt my serious health problems were mostly behind me, and I had regained most of my strength that I had before the nine hours of surgery for the kidney stones and TURP. I was also thankful that no cancer was found in my prostate. This was definitely miracle number one. I just didn't know what was looming in my near future concerning my health.

Miracle Number Two:

December 2, 2018 was a day that changed my life forever. My alarm clock sounded off, I awoke early, about 5:30 am. I had my day planned out to drive my old 1978 green and silver Chevrolet Bonanza truck with a camper shell on the back to the US # 1 Metro Flea Market, located at 3500 US 1, Augusta Highway, West Columbia, South Carolina. My plans were to rent, and set up a display of items I had for sale on a flea market table, and work on wrist watches for my regular customers, as well as sell some watches, and a few other household items and tools. I always looked forward to walking around early in the morning at the flea market and talking to my friends, and looking at the other vender's merchandise; especially if I found wrist watches or antique tools to purchase at a deal either to collect or to resell. I have always been fond of antique wood working tools made in the late 1800's and early 1900's era, and finding vintage automatic, as well as the older wind up and quartz wristwatches. On this particular morning, I ate breakfast from the food truck named The Crazy Pineapple. I ordered a BLT sandwich with extra mayonnaise, and regular caffeine coffee with lots of cream and sugar. I've always like my coffee strong and sweet. The breakfast was very good, but as soon as I finished eating, I began to feel sick on my stomach. I walked to the rest room, and immediately had a bowel movement. While having the bowel movement, I noticed some severe symptoms that seemed totally fearful and odd. I was wet with sweat from the top of my head to the top portion of my upper legs. My fingers and feet were ice cold and tingling; almost as if my fingers and feet were going to sleep and getting numb. I looked at the tips of my fingers, and they had lost some of the pink color I normally have; they were turning white. I had the common signs of a heart attack, but I had no pain. I had an aching sensation in my chest and arms that was spreading to my neck, jaw, and upper back. I was also getting lightheaded and dizzy. It was at that moment, still in the restroom that I knew for certain I was having a heart attack. It never occurred to me at that point that I might not survive. As quick as I could, I walked back to my rental table at the flea market, which was about one hundred feet away from the rest room, lay down on top of the table, and grabbed a cardboard box to put under my head for a pillow. I didn't care what people might think, with being stretched out on top of a flea market rental table; I just knew at that point in time, if I were to have a chance to survive, I had to keep extremely calm. I handed my cell phone to the man who had rented a table to by left and told him, "Call 911 right now; I'm having a heart attack." He called, and the ambulance arrived in less than ten minutes. I remember seeing some of my friends, curious of course, and gathering around me lying on the top of the table which measured four feet by eight feet to see what was happening.

The ambulance team loaded me quickly and began to go to work on me before the ambulance moved from that location at the flea market. I figured I was about five miles from the hospital, and I was still talking and thinking pretty clearly at the time. One of the medical ambulance team members asked me if I had taken any aspirin, and I told him I had taken one baby aspirin, and my blood pressure medication before I left home about 6 am. He gave me 3 more and told me to chew them up. Another man on the ambulance team gave me a shot in my right arm to help stop the heart attack. An EKG was run while in route, and all of this information was transferred to Lexington Medical Center via Internet from the ambulance. I was certainly impressed with the team work of these professionals. Upon arrival at the hospital, I was taken straight to the surgery cath lab located close to the emergency room. A critical care team was already in place there in the cath lab surgery room waiting for my arrival, and they went into motion extremely fast. My doctor did a cath on me through my right groin, and immediately began to install 3 ceramic stints in the lower left side of my heart. I remember a nurse or staff member trying to get me to sign some papers, but my doctor told her, "That can wait, we need to try to save his life right now!" She left without the signing of the papers. I remained awake and knew step by step what was happening to me. The heart doctor and care team were great, with clear instructions to me as to what they were doing to me, and what was happening to me. One of my arteries was blocked 100%, another was blocked 90%, and the third was blocked 85%. The left ventricle is one of four chambers of the heart. It is located in the bottom left portion of the heart below the left atrium, separated by the mitral valve. As the heart contracts, blood eventually flows back into the left atrium, and then through the mitral valve, whereupon it next enters the left ventricle. All of these blockages were in my left ventricle of my heart, which is the sector of the heart that is famous for the widow maker. On the big screen above me, my doctor showed me where I had a previous heart attack he thought about 7 or 8 years ago in the same area. He called this a silent heart attack, because I didn't even know I had one. Blood vessels had naturally by-passed this area, and my doctor told me there was nothing he could do to help that situation get any better than it already was. I can remember my doctor looking down at me while I was still there in the cath lab, and saying: "Mr. Davis, you just survived the widow maker." He told me later that if I had been about ten minutes more in time getting to the hospital, I may not have survived. At that time, I really didn't even know what a widow maker was.

Soon I was moved from the cath lab to a hospital room. I felt good, but was exhausted. Two days later my blood pressure crashed down to 55/20 and set off an emergency code alarm. I almost passed out and was going into cardiac arrest. The nurses came running into my room fast, and gave me meds in my IV to bring my blood pressure back up. That same day, my heart doctor came in my hospital room and told me he wanted to take me to surgery and install a pacemaker and combination defibrillator to help regulate my heart. At that time I didn't know that my heart was pumping about 30% of the blood volume of a normal healthy heart. I went to surgery late the next afternoon, and everything went well. Four days later I was discharged from the hospital and went home. This was Miracle Number Two.

Miracle Number Three:

I felt pretty good at home for the first two days. On the third day I began to have trouble breathing. On the fourth day, I could barely breath and had the death rattles when I tried to breath. My ministry experience in the past had taught me that time would be limited for life unless I acted fast to get professional help with the fluid build up. The only way I could rest was sitting up in a chair, and only then for about fifteen minutes at a time. Sleeping was out of the question. At this point, this was the first time that I thought I may just not make it, and could actually die from the complications from the widow maker. Back to the hospital I go. When I arrived at the hospital I went to a room in the ER almost immediately. Over six liters of fluid were pulled off of me in two days using Lasix (furosemide) which is an anthranilic acid derivative that is used as a strong diuretic to treat excessive fluid accumulation (edema) caused by congestive heart failure, liver failure, renal failure, and nephritic syndrome. I've also learned that Lasix may also be used with antihypertensive drugs to control high blood pressure (hypertension). I was transferred to a room on the cardiac heart floor of the hospital and stayed in the Lexington Medical Center hospital another four days before being discharged to go back home.

Again, I felt pretty good at home. I was looking forward to the Christmas holidays. My cousin Carolyn put up and decorated a beautiful Christmas tree with colorful blinking lights. I looked forward to every meal, and was thankful that I didn't have to eat hospital food any longer. I believed that my heart would heal, get back to near normal, and I would get strong enough to do the things in life that I always enjoyed. Carolyn owns an estate sale company called Estate Sales Supreme, LLC. She liquidates the contents of the home by running a tag sale that is open to the public, usually on weekends. She had a sale under contract near Lexington, South Carolina, and another one under contract in the Irmo, South Carolina area. I felt strong enough to help her with the estate sales. At least I could sit and write sales tickets, and talk to the customers. The last of December and the first part of January were pretty good. I felt that I wasn't getting much stronger, but I also felt and believed that I was certainly holding my own. This healing, in my mind, would take more time than I had originally expected. Miracle Number Three was to be happily at home from the hospital, and somewhat stable with my health.

Miracle Number Four:

By the first week of February, 2019, I knew something was really wrong, but I didn't know what it was. I felt sick just about all of the time. I began to vomit more and more, and by February 9th the vomiting was constant, day and night. I couldn't even tolerate toothpaste in my mouth. So, on February 11th I went back to the ER at Lexington Medical Center. After about 6 hours in the ER, the doctor decided to admit me. I told him that I thought my gall bladder could possibly be the problem, since I could not keep any food down. Counting my heart doctor, there were five doctors that were checking on me. Each doctor was a specialist in his or her profession. All of the doctors except one (the doctor who would be doing the gall bladder surgery) decided that it was certainly my gall bladder that was causing the problem. Yes, there were some small stones in my gall bladder, but as the surgeon told me, "Jimmy, many of the people walking out there in the hall probably have more gall stones in their gall bladder than you do." The general consensus of most of the doctors treating me was, "Take his gall bladder out, and he will be fine!" The gall bladder surgeon came back into my room on the tenth day of my hospital stay and told me that my problem was totally my heart failure, not my gall bladder. My congestive heart failure, due to complications after the heart attack, was causing all of my internal organs to shut down. Even my skin was turning a different color, and I was as white as a ghost. I had lost forty pounds of weight since my heart attack on December 2, 2018, until February 27, 2019. The surgeon refused to do surgery, and thus he saved my life. I feel like I would have certainly died during surgery if that had happened. The gall bladder surgeon convinced my heart doctor, and the other attending doctors of the real problem, and so my heart doctor called MUSC at Charleston South Carolina to try to get me a bed there in ICU. The wait was on, and three days later, MUSC called Lexington Medical Center and told my doctor that they could not accept my supplemental insurance; therefore, I could not be transferred to MUSC. Who would ever think that Blue Cross Blue Shield Insurance Company would not be accepted by a major hospital in their home state of South Carolina. I felt like 3 days had been totally wasted. A call was then made to the Heart Center at Prisma Richland Hospital, and they immediately accepted my case. Even my insurance was accepted this time. I was transferred to Richland Heart Center ICU by ambulance, on March 1, 2019, after spending nineteen days in the Lexington Medical Center Hospital, with everyone just going around and around in circles, and guessing what my real problem was. Miracle Number Four was that all the doctors at Lexington Medical Center finally decided together not to remove my gall bladder. I would learn just a few days later that I would probably not have survived that surgery.

Miracles Number Five and Six: Two Miracles before my birth:

My father, Melvin Julius Davis, born in 1921, was drafted in the Navy in World War II. He had graduated from Norway High School, in the small town of Norway, South Carolina, located on Highway 321 south of Columbia, and was planning on either a farming or a business career. He was farming on the family farm when he got the draft notice. While serving in the US Navy, his ship was docked at Norfolk Navy Yard in Virginia. My father's mother, Pearl Hutto Davis, became critically ill, and my father begged and begged his commanding officer for a ten day shore leave to go back to his home, which at that time was in Columbia, South Carolina, to check on his mother, my grandmother. The officer finally but reluctantly agreed, and allowed him to go home on leave. My grandmother was already admitted as a patient in the old Columbia Hospital in Columbia, South Carolina when my father arrived back home. Well, as things go for the good, and by the grace of God, even though everyone expected my grandmother to die, she did not, but instead recovered from her illness, and returned to her home in Columbia. I never did know why she was admitted to the hospital during World War II, but in 1965, about twenty years later, she died of complications from heart failure and heart disease. My father returned to Virginia during the War to get back on the ship and continue his duty in the war. When he arrived at the Navy yard in Virginia, his commanding officer assigned him to another ship, the USS Achomawi (ATF-148). The USS Achomawi was a Navajo-class fleet ocean tug in the service of the United States Navy, named after the Achomawi tribe of Native Americans. She was laid down as Achomawi (AT-148) on January 15, 1944, at Charleston, South Carolina by Charleston Shipbuilding and Drydock. Launched on June 14, 1944, sponsored by Mrs. J. F. Veronee, and commissioned on November 11, 1944, with Lieutenant R. H. Teter in command. The tug departed Charleston on November 28, bound for the Chesapeake Bay for shakedown training. She then entered the Norfolk Navy Yard, Portsmouth, Virginia for post-shakedown availability. My father joined the crew of the USS Achomawi at Norfolk, Virginia. The ship towed from two to three barges of military ammo at a time to the United States Army troops during World War II. Once my father told me that during a storm, one of the barges loaded with ammo came unhooked with the tow cable from the

USS Achomawi, and they had to blow up the barge, sinking it in the ocean, to keep the ammo from running into another ship or being captured by the enemy. He talked very little about the war, but this was a story he was proud of, since he helped in shooting the barge and watching it blow up. Upon arrival to get back on his ship after his mother's stay in the hospital, when my father asked his commanding officer why he was being assigned to another ship, the USS Achomawi, the answer was, "The ship you were assigned to was destroyed by the Japanese, and you are the only survivor!" What happened to the USS Achomawi? The Achomawi was removed from the reserve fleet in June of 1987, and towed to Bethlehem Shipyard for repairs. She returned from the shipyard the following month. In 1991, the ship was sold to the government of Taiwan, where she entered service with the Republic of China Navy as *Tatung* ATF-554. My father served on the USS Achomawi until his discharge from the Navy. This first pre-birth miracle is a testimony to my birth and my destiny that was to come. Wow!, (miracle number five). Had my father not been allowed to return to Columbia, South Carolina to check on his mother, I would not have even been born. God is good, and he knows His people even before birth. My father served our country well and was awarded The American Area Medal, the Asiatic-Pacific Medal, and the World War II Victory Medal. He was trained at Camp Peary, Virginia and Fort Pierce, Florida, but I suspect his real training was doing his daily duty serving our country. He died in 1993 from complications about two weeks after he had a heart attack.

Another pre-birth miracle (miracle number six) happened in the month of July 1952, the same year I was born. My birth date is September 26, 1952. My father was trying his luck at farming, in the Norway and Blackville, South Carolina areas. Back then, this was a very poor way of attempting to make a living, and he was a share-cropper to boot. He was returning from the South Carolina State Farmer's Market after selling a pickup truck load of watermelons. My mother, Viola Idelle Whitaker Davis, born in 1926, seven months pregnant with me at the time, and my sister, born in 1949, were both in the front cab of the truck with my father. As they were driving through the town of Swansea, South Carolina, southbound, returning to Norway, South Carolina, a drunk driver smashed into the side of the pickup truck on my mother's, or passenger's side, of the truck. This fluke T-bone accident totally destroyed the truck and it rolled over in the middle of highway at the intersection of highway 321 and highway 6. My father immediately kicked out the front windshield of the truck so the three of them could exit the truck through the opening of the windshield. My mother told me that the next day she was so sore in her stomach area that she went to the doctor to find out if she was losing her baby: me! Of course, there were no vehicle seatbelts laws in 1952. After her checkup at the doctor, he looked at her and said, "You can't kill him, he's a tough one!" Even though I had not been born yet, God knew me before the foundation of the world, and I can count and praise Him for these two miracles before my birth.

Miracle Number Seven:

I am considering miracle number seven to be all the extensive testing that I endured before the LVAD surgery. By March 2, 2019, I was very ill, and my heart was pumping only about twenty percent of the blood a normal healthy heart pumps. God was with me all the way, and everything I had to endure seemed to be another part of a much greater plan. After being transferred from the Lexington Medical Center to the Prisma Richland Heart Center, I immediately began a series of testing to find out if I could even qualify for the LVAD system. My insurance agent assigned to my case from Blue Cross Blue Shield came to see me and asked me some questions. She looked straight at me and asked me what were my plans. I thought that to be a bit funny considering the shape I was in, but I thought fast and said. "I actually have two plans. I have plan A, and I have plan B. Plan A, I told her, was for her to agree with me and agree to allow my insurance to pay for the upcoming procedure; and I would go through the surgery to implant the LVAD. I would get well, and lead a somewhat normal life." She said, "Then what is your plan B?" I said, "Plan B is that I do not have the surgery and I die right here in the hospital, or back at home, and I live with Jesus in heaven for eternity." I told her, "I'm okay with either plan, I'm a winner either way this goes." I knew I had won her over to my side, because she gave me a complimentary umbrella and smiled as she left the room. This nice lady would visit me again after the surgery, and retell me the uncommon story she said she was fortunate to hear.

I would endure a colonoscopy, which is an exam used to detect changes or abnormalities in the large intestine (colon) and rectum. My first colonoscopy was done when I was fifty years old, so I knew what to expect. During a colonoscopy, a long, flexible tube (colonoscope) is inserted into the rectum. A tiny video camera at the tip of the tube allows the doctor to view the inside of the entire colon. I had two polyps, which were removed during the process of this procedure. I was awake during part of this exam, and believe me, that's no fun to be awake during this procedure.

I would endure an Endocopy, which is the insertion of a long, thin tube directly into the body to observe an internal organ or tissue in detail. It can also be used to carry out other tasks including imaging and minor surgery. Endoscopes are minimally invasive and can be inserted into the openings of the body such as the mouth. My endoscope was inserted down my throat, esophagus, and into my stomach looking for ulcers, and any sign of cancer. My test went great, as expected, and nothing was found that would prevent the LVAD surgery.

I would endure a long thick needle inserted into my liver for the purpose of a biopsy. A liver biopsy is a procedure in which a needle is inserted directly into the liver to collect a tissue sample. I was awake during this procedure. The tissue is then analyzed in a laboratory to help doctors diagnose a variety of disorders and diseases in the liver. Again, that test went well, but the test did show that I had some degree of liver failure at the time, due to my heart not pumping a normal volume of blood. Also, I was told that I had stage five kidney failure, yet I had no problems with urination.

I endured multiple CT scans from the top of my head to the bottom of my legs. My brain was also scanned, but the test came back that I had none (lol). My kidneys and bladder were scanned (no kidney stones this time). The doctors looked all over my body for signs of any type of cancer or abnormalities. My teeth were x-rayed for any sign of infection, or abscess. My lungs and other organs were x-rayed. All was looking great with the testing, but I was steadily getting sicker and sicker every hour of the day.

I endured a barium swallow test (Cine esophagram, swallowing study, Esophagography). This study is a special type of imaging test that uses barium and x-rays to create images of your upper gastrointestinal (GI) tract. Your upper GI tract includes the back of your mouth and throat (pharynx) and your esophagus. I was so weak, I could barely stand up for the x-rays for this procedure.

A medical device called a Swan-Ganz was inserted into my neck and went into my heart for evaluation purposes of my heart. Swan-Ganz is a right heart catheterization. It's called Swan because it looks sort of like a bird called a Swan. Swan-Ganz catheterization is the passing of a thin tube (catheter) into the right side of the heart, and the arteries leading to the lungs. It is done to monitor the heart's function and blood flow and pressures in and around the heart. This procedure was not new to me, because while a patient at Lexington Medical Center, I had this done during that time of hospitalization. The first time this was done, the doctor doing the procedure accidentally crushed the silver wrapped tube going into my neck, and I had to go back to the operation room and have it done again. I was awake during these procedures. The doctors and nurses can use the swan device to read pressures in your heart and veins, as well as inject medication directly into your veins; so this was actually a blessing that I didn't have to get a needle stuck in my arm every few hours for some type of medication. I would have this same procedure done for a fourth time in the fall of 2019 for pre-preparation of a heart transplant. Miracle number seven was actually a series of multiple miracles designed to prepare me for the HeartMate Three LVAD system.

What is an LVAD? A left ventricular assist device, or LVAD, is a mechanical pump that is implanted inside a person's chest to help a weakened heart pump blood. Unlike a total artificial heart, the LVAD doesn't replace the heart. It just helps your heart do its job. My LVAD helped my heart pump about one gallon of blood per minute, and the titanium bearing-less pump inside my chest rotated at approximately 5200 rpms per minute. LVADs may also be used as "destination therapy." This means it is used long-term in some terminally ill people whose condition makes it impossible for them to be a candidate for a heart transplant.

Like the heart, the LVAD is a pump. It's surgically implanted just below the heart. One end is attached to the bottom of the left ventricle -- that's the chamber of the heart that pumps blood out of the heart and into the body. The other end, a tube that is attached to the pump, is attached to the aorta, the body's main artery at the top of the heart. Blood flows from the heart into the pump. When sensors within the control module, worn externally, indicate that the LVAD is full, the blood in the device is moved into the aorta. You cannot hear the pump running. Getting a blood pressure reading is a bit more difficult, and in my case, I could not feel a pulse. Recent data suggest that high blood pressure contributes to life-threatening complications such as pump thrombosis and stroke of CF-LVAD patients. When I had a heart clinic visit, my blood pressure was taken with a method called Doppler, and also the regular standard cuff blood pressure. The blood is a steady flow, just like turning on a water hose and allowing the water to flow through the hose. With LVAD patients, a tube passes from the internal pump device through the skin, usually to the right side of your stomach area. This tube, called the driveline, connects the internal pump to the external control module and power source. The driveline has seven small wires inside and is wrapped in Kevlar for added strength. The pump and its connections are implanted during open-heart surgery. A computer controller, sometimes called a system controller, a dual power pack, (in my case there were two 14 volt lithium batteries), and a reserve power pack inside the control module remain outside the body. Some models allow a person wear these external units on a belt or harness outside. The early models were more bulky than the HeartMate Three. In my case, I had the harness, but I preferred wearing a special T shirt. I had T shirts that are made especially for the HeartMate Three, so the batteries could be worn one on the left side of my waist and one on the right side of my waist, and I could wear the control module either around my neck in a leather pouch especially made for the control module, or place it either to the left or the right side just below one of the batteries. The T shirts are sold at www.lvadshirt.com, and are made of 92% polyester and 8% spandex. They are made in Poland, and the cost per shirt is approximately $85.00. The shirts are available in with white or black colors. My sister Betty Ann purchased these shirts for me the week after I had the LVAD surgery, and I remain very thankful to her. The shirts are machine washable, but I did not put them in the dryer, but instead just let them air dry. I preferred to wear the control module around my neck suspended by a thirty inch long and one inch wide collar, that resembles a dog collar, that ran through the top of the leather pouch that held the control module. For me, this allowed me more freedom, especially when getting in and our of the car or other tight places. This system was worn so close to my body that no one could tell by looking that I was an LVAD patient. At night, I just removed the collar and let it rest beside me in the bed to my right side. I had a total of cight 14 volt lithium-ion rechargeable batteries that measure 6" long, 3" wide and 1" thick each, and weigh 1 pound 2 ounces each, a charging station that charged 4 batteries at a time, and a HeartMate Three wall unit that allowed me to come off of the battery packs when needed, especially at night when sleeping. The wall unit has 3 AA batteries that have to be changed out every three months; and the spare control module needs to be charged off of the wall unit approximately every three months. There is also a red LVAD rubber bracelet that should be worn all the time. The bracelet has the emergency LVAD phone number on it; and I kept it on my carry on bag at all times. If you are an LVAD patient, you will be trained in all aspects of how to care and maintain the equipment. There is also a quick short guide available to you just in case you have to change out the control module in a emergency situation. The control module has a back-up power source of approximately fifteen minutes, in case of an emergency, and the battery packs fail. Every LVAD patient has to notify his or her local fire department, in case of an emergency electrical power outage, so the fire station can be aware that their generator may be needed to charge the LVAD batteries. Also, the electric power company is required to place a special seal on your home electric power meter stating that the power company cannot turn the electricity off at your home. In the area where I live, this is called: The White Cross Program, and it is for customers with special medical device needs. Everywhere an LVAD patient goes, he or she must carry the pouch with the two extra batteries and a spare control module. It's critical to keep these spare parts with you at all times. There are currently approximately 25,000 LVAD patients worldwide.

The following are ten points, basically common information, to remember about Left Ventricular Assist Devices (LVADs) as a rapidly evolving alternative to transplant: I found some of this information on the Internet, and pieced it together to help you if you know someone with an LVAD, or if you are an LVAD patient yourself. One thing I have learned, is: "Do not be afraid." Treat the LVAD system just as if it is just another part of your human body. Whatever your situation, rest assured that God is much greater than we are, and He is in control. I am often reminded of a favorite passage of scripture: "I

Can Do All Things Through Christ Who Strengthens Me" (Philippians 4:13). With a persistent donor shortage, and an increasing number of patients with Stage D heart failure, LVADs have been used as bridge to heart transplant for those who qualify for transplant (bridge to transplant), or as a substitute in those who do not (destination therapy). You're in this phase of Stage D if you have systolic heart failure (your heart muscle doesn't squeeze with enough force). Despite ongoing measures to increase access to donor organs, organ availability remains a major limitation to heart transplant. The current strategy for the management of refractory Stage D heart failure with reduced ejection fraction (HFrEF) patients is to initially screen for heart transplant, with destination therapy, LVADs or VADs are considered as secondary treatment for those who do not qualify. The current algorithm for screening patients for advanced heart failure therapies may need to be revisited in the near future, with a shift to considering patients initially for destination VAD and heart transplant reserved for selected patients, or as bailout therapy. VAD support offers improved quality of life and survival, compared to medical therapy, and in some cases, have two year outcomes comparable to heart transplant. There are now more LVAD implants performed per year than heart transplants (you can document this fact with an Internet search). LVAD complications persist and may have lessened enthusiasm for investigating LVAD therapy in less sick patients; however, technology continues to advance rapidly. Smaller devices, total implant ability, pulsatility, and remote monitoring are being investigated, and will broaden application of VAD technology. Clinical trials are certainly needed to determine which patients benefit most from LVAD support versus heart transplantation. LVAD technology is evolving rapidly and its accessibility is increasing when compared to heart transplant. In the future, LVADs may be considered initial therapy for Stage D heart failure, with heart transplant reserved for LVAD failures and selected patients. I'm praying as of this writing that I will become a selected patient. The downturn to this move toward heart transplant, is I realize that someone must give the ultimate sacrifice of his or her heart and life, that I may gain a healthy heart again. As of the writing of this chapter in my short book, I realize that this, as sad as it will be for that family with their loss of their loved one, it would be a separate miracle of blessing for me.

Miracle Number Eight:

For over a month prior to March 6, 2019, I was one sick puppy. I was more ready to die than I was to live. March 6, 2019 is a date I will always remember. This was the date of my major heart surgery at Prisma Richland Hospital for the LVAD system. The surgery took approximately 5.5 hours, and I was told afterward that all went well. I had lived in total misery for the past six to seven weeks. At this point, the doctors could cut off my head and I would be okay with that if it made me feel better as an end results. I had prayed that God's will be done, and I had surrendered everything in my life to Him. If it were God's will that I die and be with Him eternally, I was okay with that. I know heaven is a much better place than life here on earth. If it were God's will that I live, I would be willing to do that also. I had lots of time on my hands to consider both life and death. At this point in my life, no material things mattered any more. A home, a car, any material things I had collected and enjoyed over my life were just worthless junk, none of this mattered or was important to me anymore. As odd as this may sound, I was even willing in my mind to separate myself from any of my family members, and closest friends; because in my mind, the journey I may soon be taking into eternity was one that I would have to make totally on my own, into the outreached arms of Jesus, and into the eternal light of God. I didn't fear death, and saw that death could be a great blessing and relief. My experience as a minister was very helpful. I had stood at the bedside of many people over the years as they took their last breath, including my own mother who passed in August, 2016. Some die easy, some die hard. If I were to die, I knew in my heart it would be an easy death. I had given over to God all my past wrongs. I knew I was forgiven for everything I had ever done in my life, and like the Apostle Paul, I had been a chief of sinners. At his point in my life, death could become the greatest blessing and miracle of them all. My cousin, Carolyn prayed the same prayer I was praying, that "If it was God's will for me to live, then let me live, but if it was my time to die, she could understand that also." As we were both praying the same prayers, God already had His perfect team of professionals ready and in place to extend my life. I couldn't tell you how many churches and people were praying for me, but somehow I felt all of this prayer power in my heart, and knowing this was a great help to me during this greatest time of need.

The day before my surgery, March 5, 2019, I was determined to take a shower, knowing it would be my last one for awhile. I managed to cut my hair all by myself (I wanted my hair to be short and easy to care for after the surgery, so I cut it extremely short), and also cut my toenails and fingernails, and took a shower. Boy was I exhausted after that ordeal. I could barely wait to get back in that hospital bed!

I don't even remember going from the hospital room to the operating room. I think the strong pre-surgery pain meds were already kicking in. The doctor prepared my family members as to what to expect after the surgery. My doctor said they could expect to see me very pale and looking almost like death after the surgery. I was told a few days later that I actually looked better after the surgery than I did before. My color was coming back to normal, my skin had a pinkish tone again. My blood was flowing again. Wow, what a surprise! Anyway, I lost about three days of memory after the heart surgery, drifting in and out of sleep. I was told later by some of my visitors that I said many stupid things that made no sense. I remember seeing what I thought at the time was the dark shadow of someone climbing up and down, and across the walls of my hospital room. The shadow looked like an older woman dressed in light gray stringy clothes. She had long dark gray hair. The image I have of this was the creature was scurrying across the wall from one side of the room to the other. What ever it was, it did not speak to me or try to get close to me. Sometimes it would stay in a corner and just watch. In my mind this was very real at the time. I remember having a similar experience in 1979 when I broke my right femur bone and was in the hospital after surgery and taking some heavy duty pain medications. My memory of that experience was of a Victorian era military officer in full uniform standing in the doorway of my hospital room. He had a black hat on his head, and along with his deep royal blue uniform, he had bright gold tassels on his shoulders. Of course that was just an image in my mind due to the pain medication, I believed. The pain after the LVAD surgery was managed, but I remember at times it was indeed pretty tough.

After the surgery for the implant of the LVAD, I began to cry uncontrollably for no known reason. I could be sitting up in the hospital chair, or in the hospital bed, perfectly happy, and just burst out in uncontrolled crying, even with real tears. I couldn't really speak plain thoughts because I couldn't stop crying. My family members were there for me with full support. I thought some of the crying could be due to some of the strong medications I was on, and perhaps it was, or even some form of depression I was going through. My experience in life had taught me that depression is a well-documented adverse effect of many surgical procedures, yet many surgeons fail to warn patients about their risks, and treatment facilities do not routinely screen patients for postoperative depression. Especially strong correlations exist between postoperative depression and heart surgery, so if you cry without being able to control your crying, and are somewhat depressed after a major surgery, you can rest assured that you are not alone. I found myself dwelling on everything that I figured was wrong in my life, past and present, and that made the crying worse. For example, my youngest son had quadruple by-pass heart surgery about a month after I got home from the rehab center. Heart disease runs in my family. He was forty one years old, and he had some of the same experiences with uncontrollable crying. I've found this is somewhat common, and even though I didn't feel depressed, I was certainly more prone to postoperative depression than I was aware of. The crying got better after a few months, and now a few years have passed and I don't do the crying anymore. I did not take any medication for this situation, but instead just rode it out until it got better.

After about a week in ICU and then a few days in the Multery Suite at Prisma Richland Hospital, I was transferred to a nearby rehab center. May I say, the nurses who worked in the ICU and Multery Suite were wonderful. I was determined to ace this and go home as quickly as possible. However, on the first morning of my stay in the rehab center, I drank a cup of caffeine coffee, and my LVAD control module sounded off it's first emergency alarm. It beeps very loud if something is wrong. Also, to make things worse, I was shocked with what I can only describe as a bolt of lightening from the defibrillator part of my pacemaker. If you've ever had this happen to you, then you know that's a barrel of fun (loll). Even my eyes were seeing strange lights from this jolt of electrical current. I may add that this charge of electricity from my defibrillator part of the pacemaker fired off three times, and was adjusted by the professionals who checked the unit to get it back into reasonable control settings. The nurse in charge at the rehab center called an ambulance, and instead of sending me to the LVAD heart clinic, she sent me to the emergency room. Of course the LVAD doctor had to be called to go to the emergency room, and after seven hours in the emergency room, and test after test, the conclusion was the caffeine in the coffee was too strong, and it set off the alarm. I didn't have any more coffee during my stay there, but as time went on, I found that I can tolerate some caffeine. I mostly drink purified water, but I do love Southern Sweet Tea with a touch of lemon.

The two workout exercise and therapy sessions each day at the rehab center helped me to build my strength. I also enjoyed the group therapy, and meeting others who were patients at the rehab center. At first, I couldn't even stand up by myself, I was so weak. A rehab worker had to grab me at the back of my pants or belt and pull me up out of the wheel chair. One of the things I did everyday was to foot peddle my way around the halls in my wheelchair to help build strength in my lower and upper legs.

After open heart surgery, the patient is not allowed for a few weeks, to use his or her hands to push the body into a stand up position. I learned quickly that it takes great strength in the legs to make this move without the help of pushing up with my arms. I placed a three inch thick pad in my wheelchair seat that helped me to sit higher in the wheelchair, thus shortening the distance I needed to fully stand. One setback I had during my stay in rehab was I got a stomach virus that was going around in the facility. This horrible stomach virus lasted about six days. That was tough on top of tough, since I was either on battery power with two fourteen lithium volt batteries, or on the wall power cable which could only reach about twenty-five feet. Sometimes, during this stomach virus, I had to act fast to get to the restroom in time, and I did have a few accidents that the nurse's aid had to clean up. Not too proud of that, but everyone was super nice and understanding. During my stay at the rehab center, it was Spring time, and I could look out my window each day and watch the birds and the leaves getting stronger and greener on the trees. I didn't know I had so many friends. Many came to visit, and I was blessed by them all. After twelve days of rehab, I rang the "I'm Going Home bell" and went home.

I had a long way to go with healing at home. I could barely get in and out of bed by myself. I couldn't drive until the doctor gave me the okay to drive (I sneaked a few times with my driving, lol). My days of activity were limited at first, but I could feel myself getting stronger day-by-day, and week-by-week. A simple cough or sneeze can be extremely painful in the chest area after major heart surgery. I was good at learning to not lift heavy objects, because I knew this could damage my rib area that was wired back together after the surgery. Doctor's orders were not to life over five pounds. Soon, I was able to go back to the flea markets and enjoy doing some of the things I loved to do. Miracle number eight was the actual LVAD surgery, the wonderful and fully dedicated professional people who were responsible and well trained to make this happen, as well as the hospital facilities and the rehab and healing that followed directly after.

What can you expect when the true healing begins? When I arrived at the clinic each time, after a quick registration, my weight was always checked, and blood was always drawn. It took a bit of getting use to, but was just part of the overall project of monitoring my health. My labs were usually great, an aspect I am really proud of. My trips to the LVAD clinic continued to be easier and easier, and soon I was changing the drive-line bandage once a week instead of every day. It is yours or perhaps a family member or close friend's responsibility to order the daily or weekly bandage dressings and supplies you will require. Since I was changing the drive line bandage once each week, instead of daily, I ordered the weekly bandage kits from Alere Home Montoring Products located in Livermore, California. If you run short, you can always purchase these bandage kits on the Internet, but the cost is pretty high. The weekly maintenance kits # EEDM190 include: a procedural insert, two masks, two hand sanitizers, two pair of gloves, two saline wipes, two skin protectants, two antiseptic applicators, an antimicrobial dressing, one closure piece, one SorbaView shield dressing (with a see through window), and one Foley cathier/driveline securement, as well as one wrap. I found it is best to change the cathier/driveline securement at least twice each week, so my skin was not irritated as much. I switched back and forth with different styles, sometimes using the double strap cath grip # 51300NS, and sometimes using the single grip strap that came with the weekly maintenance kit. The double strap grip is a lot more secure, but it is also larger and irritated my skin more. Also, you will be required to order the 2 x 2 dressing that goes directly over the driveline area, under the outer bandage, where it enters your stomach area. I found the DeRoyal brand was best if that brand can be found. The DeRoyal brand is # 46-TD22, Algidex Trach Dressing. The reason I prefer this dressing is because it has a slit and round hole in the middle that fits firmly over the driveline where it entered my body. All of the dressings and materials you will require come with easy to follow instructions and great general information. My personal health insurance company only allowed me to order five of the weekly driveline management systems at a time, so it's always good to order a few weeks before you actually run out of these supplies, since sometimes the order may be placed on a company back-order status, and you are left waiting and wondering when the supplies you desperately need will arrive. Usually the LVAD clinic you attend for regular checkups can spare a few supplies to you in an emergency situation. It is also good to carefully look at the driveline area, and if you should ever notice something that is not normal, or an infection in that area, call the LVAD clinic immediately. If you are an LVAD patient, you must be trained as to the proper procedure of changing the driveline bandage. Another person, maybe a family member, or friend, must also be trained, so being an LVAD patient is actually a joint venture, and not a solo lifestyle. Having the great fortune and blessing of an LVAD system is also extremely costly. In the year 2019, my insurance company and Medicare were billed almost $1,300,000.00 for the procedures, surgeries, medications, and supplies needed. With an LVAD HeartMate Three, three ceramic stints in my heart area, and a combination pace maker and defibrillator, I'm well on my way to becoming a true bionic man.

My meds have changed a few times after surgery, especially some of the blood pressure medications. The cost of meds continue to climb, and I noticed recently that my blood pressure medication alone is costing $563.00 per month. I've been very fortunate that my health insurance pays for most of my medications, and I have only a very low co-pay out of pocket. I've had a few alarms from the control module, but nothing really serious. If your blood pressure gets too high or too low, an alarm will sound. As of this part of the writing of my story, April, 2020, I feel almost as strong as I did before the major heart attack in December 2018. I can't move a refrigerator by myself, but I can easily pick up a 50 pound bag of dog food, or even do some light mechanic work on my vehicles.

Due to the Corona Virus, my appointment for April 20, 2020 was done by using Face Time on iPhone for the first time. I can probably expect more of these type health checkups in the future, which suits me okay, since my drive time to the LVAD clinic is approximately 1.5 hours for the round trip. My heart doctor, nurse, and nurse practioner joined in the conference. All meds are good, my doctor took me off Mag-Oxide, and my Dr. said he would call the heart clinic in Charlotte, North Carolina, and advocate for me for a heart transplant. I will need to get the transplant before I am age 70, since that is usually the cut off age for heart transplants. I have my INR checked about every 10 days to 2 weeks, and that information is faxed to the heart clinic at Prisma Richland Hospital Heart Clinic; then a pharmacy worker calls me that same day, and tells me the result. A good INR reading is between 2.0 and 3.0. Mine is usually about 2.4.

Miracle Number Nine:

I had a non invasive in situ melanoma cancer removal on my head above my right eye on Jan. 30th, 2020, and a second time March 2, 2020. Melanoma in situ is also called stage "0" melanoma. It means there are cancer cells in the top layer of skin (the epidermis). The melanoma cells are all contained in the area in which they started to develop, and have not grown into deeper layers of the skin, or spread to any glands. Some doctors call in situ cancers pre cancer. My plastic surgeon doctor missed a small piece of it the first time. I have a light scar there near my hairline about three inches long, but you know, the scars you have on your body just proof you have lived. I got blessed because I had a great doctor with lots of experience, who is also a professor with the University of South Carolina Medical School. He even participated in the first heart transplant in the state of Arizona when he was a med student there in Arizona. All patients to be considered for a heart transplant have to be cancer free before the transplant surgery. Therefore I consider this surgery and healing my miracle number nine.

What can you expect after the LVAD transplant? First, lots of appointments with doctors, nurses, and frequent testing. Every time I go to the LVAD clinic I am hooked up to a diagnostic machine and checked for the condition of the equipment, and what, if any critical and recent information is stored in the control module. Sometimes, I get a pacemaker and defibrillator check during my normal clinic visit. Sometimes I am asked to walk for six minutes around the hall at the clinic to see if I am stable on my feet. I've been told that I am one of the fastest walkers they have who have LVAD units. As stated earlier, complete blood work for the lab is always standard.

At home, taking a bath or shower is a chore. Of course, swimming is out of the question, but just taking a shower can wear you down physically. I have a special two compartment water proof case that holds the control module and the two 14 volt batteries. This special shower case has a see through window at the top so you can still see the control module if it were to sound an alarm. I wear the water proof case around my neck attached to a wide strap, and take a shower. Immediately after the shower, I change my weekly driveline bandage; so I usually do not take more than one full shower a week. The other days are sponge off baths, and washing my hair in the sink. I know these daily things seem to be simple, but believe me, your life will really change after an LVAD.

I was told by my doctors to never run a vacuum cleaner because the static electricity could interfere with the electronics of the LVAD. That's fine with me, but I have been told that I can still do some work and push a broom. Using a microwave seems to be okay. Another thing to be careful of after the LVAD implant is to be very careful standing up quickly or making sudden moves like twisting too quickly. I've gotten dizzy a few times standing up too quick from a chair or getting out of bed in the morning to quick. Keep your blinders on, just like an old plow mule has blinders on his head in the field, and always look forward instead of looking back or side to side. Always looking forward reduces dizzy spells. It is also advisable to sleep on your back instead of other positions. I have found that if I turn to my left side to sleep, I cannot, due to a light pain near my heart area where the titanium pump is resting beside my heart. Sometimes, I do sleep on my right side, but care has to be taken with the driveline bandage site and the driveline itself.

Also, expect that with the blood thinners, if you accidentally cut or nick your skin, you may bleed for hours, or even need to go to the ER for treatment. Even a small nick on your hand can continue to bleed until it finally begins to clot. I've been fortunate so far with very few minor cuts and bruises.

Here is a list of my medications, and perhaps some you can expect to take daily after having an LVAD: Your list may or may not include these medications.

Mag-Oxide 400mg (Stop as of 4-20-2020)--clinic doctor stopped this one.

Carvedilol (Coreg) 6.25mg for blood pressure 1 am and 1 pm. (helps to dilate (keep open) blood vessels around the heart).

Aspirin 81 coated (Morning) for heart, also a mild blood thinner.

Bumetanide (Bumex) 1MG as needed for fluid build up.

Potassium Chloride (Klor-Con) 20 mEq--take one when take Bumetanide 1MG as needed for fluid build up (supplement).

Entresto (Sacubitril-valsartan) 97mg/103mg combination med (Blood Pressure) take 1 am and 1 pm.

Rosuvastatin 20mg (Crestor), 1 every evening For cholesterol.

Side Effects of Crestor: mild memory problems or confusion.

Ondansetron HCL 4mg (Zofran) as needed for nausea.

Gabapentin (Neurontin) 100mg--take as needed for joint pain usually pm if needed.

Pantoprazole (Protonix) 4OMG (Evening) Acid Reflux.

Quetiapine Fumarate (Seroquel) 25mg (Evening) for Mood.

Warfarin (Coumadin) 2MG (I take 2 tablets on Sun., Mon. Wed. & Friday), I take 3 Tablets on Tues, Thurs, Sat. (blood thinner). Note: Warfarin is the only blood thinner a person can take after LVAD. INR has to be checked approximately every ten days to two weeks with a finger prick. Full labs are usually drawn every month to six weeks.

Miracle Number Ten:

I believe that God had all the professional health care people, and facilities already in place for my heart transplant. About July of 2020, I talked to my LVAD team at a regular scheduled checkup about the possibility of getting a heart transplant. My doctors indicated they would advocate for me. About a month later I got a phone call from Advent Health Transplant Center in Orlando Florida. After several questions on the phone, the transplant coordinator asked if I would be willing to come to Orlando to be evaluated for a heart transplant. So, in August of 2020, my sister and I traveled to Orlando for four days of intense evaluation. I met with nurses, doctors, exam technicians, and endured various test to prepare me for what was to come. I was approved the next week after all the test came back, so now I just have to be patient and prayerfully wait.

On September 14, I moved to Orlando and booked a room in an Extended Stay America in Maitland, Florida, about seven miles away from Advent Health, which is located in downtown Orlando. I chose the ESA because it has a small kitchen, and I knew that I would have to do some of my own cooking during the stay, which I did not know how long the wait would be. It turned out that I would stay there a full three months until the perfect miracle heart became available. During the first three months of my stay, I went through a lot of checkups and testing again, and was admitted to Advent Health hospital once for seven days to adjust my LVAD system, which was showing low flow and becoming somewhat unstable. During this wait, I also got two false starts for a donor heart. I went to Rapid In And Out twice and was there waiting to go into surgery, but both times the nurse came in and told me that the donor heart was not a perfect match. Once, the donor heart was from a prisoner, and I had to sign papers indicating that I agreed to accept that donor heart, but unfortunately, that heart did not match. Even though I was somewhat disappointed, I knew that God was in charge, not me, so again, I was learning to be patient and wait.

About 7:30am on the morning of December 17, 2020, my cousin Carolyn was sitting in our den praying. She asked God to show her a miracle that day, that I would soon get my heart transplant. Carolyn always sees red birds (Cardinals) as a sign that something good is about to happen. That morning, she prayed not to just see one or two Cardinals, but she told God in prayer that she would love to see an entire flock of Cardinals. After her prayer, she looked out of our home toward the pear tree that my grandmother planted in 1939, and she saw eight Cardinals fluttering around the pear tree. She figured that I would soon be transplanted. In the Bible, the number eight is a meaning for "a new beginning." I got the call from my coordinator at Advent Health that same day, December 17, 2020, about 9:30am.

By 10:30am I was back in Rapid In And Out at Advent Health Transplant Center. I felt at ease this time, that today was the day, and everything felt like it was in place for the perfect donor heart. I was prepped for surgery and by 2pm as I was being wheeled down the hall to the OR, my lights went out in deep sleep. I would wake up in ICU about two days later. The surgery for my heart transplant took from 2pm until 12am. I would learn later that my cousin Carolyn felt two heavy thumps in her own heart at 7:56pm on the night of December 17. She asked me about a week later to find out the time the donor heart started beating. I asked one of my nurses to look in my chart, and she indicated that my new heart began beating at 7:56pm, and it was pumping approximately seven liters of blood a minute.

I was in ICU for at least five days. I had eight tubes in my chest, and a 24 gauge Foley catheter. My weight soured up to approximately 300 pounds because of all the fluids they were pumping into my body. My heart surgeon came in one day and told me that he had transplanted a young strong heart into me that he would be proud to transplant into any of his family members if they needed a heart. The pain was being managed somewhat, but not totally. Dreams were unreal because of all the medications to manage the pain. I kept dreaming of a burgundy wall that kept changing like moving stones full of statues. I dreamed also of white ships moving through a channel of rocks in a salty sea. The nurses would move me to the chair every day to prevent infections, and sometimes leave me in the chair for up to 14 hours at a time. Finally I was moved out of ICU to the seventh floor on the Ginsburg Tower at Advent Health. All the meds changed from the LVAD to new meds after my heart transplant.

My total stay in the hospital was 21 days after transplant. All of the doctors and professional nurses and exam teams were absolutely wonderful. On December 24, I had a mild setback becoming constipated from the medication. I was given laxatives, and on

Christmas day, 2020, I had the shittiest Christmas I have ever had (lol), pooping 14 times that day (13 of those unfortunately in the bed). I knew I was improving, keeping a positive attitude, and I told my nurses that the only way to eat this type of elephant would be one bite at a time.

I was discharged on January 8, 2021, and my son Jason and I went back to the Extended Stay America in Maitland. I would stay there almost three more months until returning back to South Carolina. The anti-rejection drugs caused me to shake like I had Parkinson's. My son stayed with me about one month, then my sister Betty Ann came back from South Carolina and stayed with me about five weeks. During the time my sister was staying with me, I became constipated again and had to be admitted again to the hospital for that, and medication adjustment. When my sister went back to South Carolina, my cousin Chandler came to Orlando and stayed with me about a week. He would drive me back to South Carolina. Finally, I would ease my way back into my own routine and continue the healing process. Since returning to my home in South Carolina, I have had some good days and some bad days, but my health is improving, and I'm getting stronger every month.

The last week in June, 2021 was pretty tough. I got to the point where I could not keep any food or liquids down. So, I went to the emergency room at Prisma Hospital in Columbia. I was fortunate to get the doctor on call who installed my LVAD. He called Advent-Health in Orlando, and was fortunate enough to get my assigned doctor who was treating me after my transplant. The decision was made to fly me on an air ambulance to Florida, just in case I was having some rejection of the heart. That trip billed my insurance for $79,000.00. It turned out that I had a UTI, but I still stayed a week in the hospital for treatment and testing. As of this writing, I return to Orlando once every three months for health checkups. This will eventually go to every six months, then once each year. I am thankful and grateful for my new donor heart.

Miracle Number Eleven:

This final miracle in my journey in life will be Meeting Jesus face to face in heaven and reuniting with my loved ones already there. We will be reunited not only with our own families and loved ones, but also with the people of God from all ages from eternity past. In heaven, we will all be one loving family. The immense size of the family will not matter in the infinite perfection of heaven. There will be ample opportunity for close relationships with everyone, and our eternity will be spent in just that kind of rich, unending fellowship, with God the Father, God the Son, God the Holy Spirit, and all the resident souls of heaven. If you're worried about feeling out of place in heaven, don't! Heaven will seem more like home than the greatest spot on earth to you. Heaven has been uniquely designed by a tender, loving Savior to be the place where we will live together for all eternity and enjoy Him forever. Perhaps that will give you some comfort for the final miracle in this book, which is your personal miracle of faith.

Miracle Number Twelve: Your Personal Miracle of Faith

As there were twelve Disciples of Jesus, this story is my testimony of my twelve miracles of faith. If you are not a Christian, this is how you can become a Christian. Have you ever wondered what you must do to become a Christian? The Bible has an answer that is easy to understand. My prayer for miracle number twelve is that all who read this will know the Lord Jesus Christ as personal Savior.

FIRST: You must understand your need to be saved. The Bible says you need to be saved because you are a sinner. Your sin has a penalty, and that penalty is death and eternal separation from God. You cannot save yourself. The Bible says, "all have sinned," and "the wages of sin is death" (Romans 3:23; 6:23).

SECOND: You must understand you can be saved from your sin. You can be saved because Christ died on the cross for your sins. The Bible says, "God demonstrated His love toward us, in that while we were yet sinners, Christ died for us" (Romans 5:8).

THIRD: You must understand what you need to do to be saved. The Bible says how you can be saved. Acts 3:19 says we must repent and turn away from our sins. But repentance alone is not enough. Ephesians 2:8 says that we must place our faith in Jesus Christ to be saved.

NOW: You must act if you want to be saved. God is waiting for you to "want to" and to ask Him to save you. The Bible says, "Whosoever will call upon the name of the Lord will be saved" (Romans 10:13). If you are ready to trust Christ as your Savior and Lord, invite Christ into your heart right now by praying to Him. You may pray the printed prayer here or you may word your own prayer.

"Dear Lord Jesus, I know that I am a sinner. I know you died for my sins. Right now, this very moment, I invite you into my heart to be my Savior and Lord. I willingly turn from my sin and give my life to you. Thank you for saving me. Amen."

Welcome to God's family. You have just made the greatest decision of your life. Tell a pastor or a friend, and especially your family members about your decision as soon as possible.

Letter to my heart donor family:

Dear Heart Donor Family,

I am overwhelmed as I write this letter, and cannot find the appropriate words to express my sincere gratitude for this ultimate gift of life. You also have my deepest sympathy for the loss of your loved one. No words I could possibly write could help you with the grief of your overwhelming loss. Please accept my thanks for the gift of your loved one's heart that has saved and changed my life.

Before my heart transplant on December 17, 2020, I had a heart attack in December 2018, and then three months later had an LVAD installed to assist my heart. The LVAD helped sustain my heart for one year and nine months. I was on a waiting list for a heart transplant for three months. My only hope for long term survival was a heart transplant, and I knew that someone would be giving up his or her life for me to continue to have life. As I went to heart transplant surgery, my thoughts were with you that day, and I am grateful that even in your extreme grief and pain you agreed to give me the chance of life. The heart transplant has tremendously improved my health and quality of life. I have a lot of people in my family whom I love and cherish, including two sons, and two grandsons. Family and faith are extremely important to me, and I am truly thankful.

You and your loved one are never far from my thoughts. My doctors have assured me that this heart is a perfect match for me, and so far, I have not had any rejection. I would like to learn more if you choose to contact me. Thank you for your generosity and for my gift of life.

Postscript:

May God Richly Bless You, and thank you for reading my short book--Jimmy Davis.

www.ingramcontent.com/pod-product-compliance
Lightning Source LLC
Chambersburg PA
CBHW080437220526
45465CB00009B/3321